Shiatsu Massage
An Alternative Healing Therapy

By: A.E Wilson

Printed by: CreateSpace, Amazon. Com Company (2014)

Shiatsu Massage
An Alternative Healing Therapy

By: A.E Wilson

Table of Contents

Chapter I - An Introduction to Shiatsu Massage

Massage is one of the most effective methods of relaxation. One will just have to sit back or lie down and let the practitioner weave his or her magic just by kneading those tired, knotted muscles for an hour or so.

Today, when you look at the 'menu' of a massage place, you will see and can choose from various styles of rubdowns. There's the Swedish massage, the Deep Tissue Massage and Reflexology among so many others. Perhaps, one of the most popular types is Shiatsu.

Shiatsu: More than Just a Massage

Shiatsu is an ancient Japanese art of healing. Since this is a form of healing, this was not just a simple massage that most people nowadays deem it to be. It was used to treat various health conditions such as headaches, nausea, vomiting and even psychological disorders like depression and anxiety.

In the old Eastern countries, the human body is considered to be a very powerful source of energy, or Qi. This life force must be balanced (yin and yang) and free flowing. The imbalance or blockage of the Qi will be the root cause of the disease.

Through the squeezing and tapping of muscles in Shiatsu, the blocked Qi will be released, allowing the energy to flow throughout the body once more and, in essence, heal itself. It does not just focus on the physical part of the body. It is more holistic in its healing approach.

The Role of Shiatsu in Modern Medicine

Since ancient practitioners stand by the degree of its effectiveness in healing, some medical professionals today have also attempted to do Shiatsu or use it to accompany the therapies that they have planned for their patients.

Some of the people who have tried this massage style as a mode of treatment for their ailments have said that Shiatsu is indeed very effective. Skeptics believe that, because all massages will give one a feeling of comfort, the heightened sense of well-being is more of a placebo effect rather than actual healing.

However, there are various tests and researches done today just to prove the effectiveness of Shiatsu in healing and to see if it can be used as a mode of treatment in hospitals as well.

Chapter II - History of Shiatsu Massage

The ancient healing art Shiatsu hails from Japan. The word Shiatsu is derived from the words 'shi' and 'atsu' which basically means finger pressure.

As mentioned earlier, ancient Japanese healers believed that the main cause of various diseases and its symptoms is the imbalance in the body which, in turn, is due to blocked Qi. The fingers are used to manipulate the muscles so that the energy will flow freely, allowing the body to heal on its own.

The Chinese Connection

It is very similar to the old Chinese art of Acupressure which also makes use of the fingers and the palms of the hand to massage the muscles of the body, therefore releasing the blocked Qi or energy.

Actually, some historians believe that Shiatsu was based on Acupressure. The first knowledge of the Qi is dated during the Han Dynasty (around 206BC to 220AD) when written accounts have been dug up in a tomb. Besides that, human remains which were mummified during the same time have been observed to have acupuncture needle points on the skin, which meant that they already practiced this in the past.

Invention of Shiatsu

More specifically, Shiatsu was developed from Anma, a mixture of Japanese massage and Chinese acupressure. Anma involves the application of pressure, tapping and rubbing of the body to stimulate the flow of Qi.

Tamai Tempaku is the person who is credited when it comes to the invention of the Shiatsu massage when he started it in the early 20th century. Since 1964, the government of Japan recognizes this as a legitimate medical therapy.

Schools of Shiatsu

Today, there are numerous styles of Shiatsu. However, the Namikoshi System and the Zen Shiatsu are the two most famous. These two are considered to be 'authentic' medical modes of treatment since it incorporated the scientific knowledge, especially anatomy and physiology.

The Japan Shiatsu College was founded by Tokujiro Namikoshi in the '40s. By applying his knowledge in anatomy and physiology to the ancient knowledge, Shiatsu became more justifiable as an effective mode of treatment. Marilyn Monroe was a patient of his, helping him to be accepted by the medical world in the west.

Zen Shiatsu is very similar to Namikoshi's System except that it focuses more on psychological disorders. Shizuto Masunaga, its founder, is a psychologist. He integrated the ancient theories of pressure points and neurology in this form of Shiatsu.

Chapter III - Shiatsu and Qi (The Shiatsu Meridians)

As mentioned in the first chapter, Shiatsu is more than just rubbing and tapping the muscles for healing and achievement of wellness. Since this is a holistic type of therapy, there are more elements of Shiatsu which must be known and understood.

Qi – the Living Energy

When learning Shiatsu, the most important lesson which must be focused on is the theory of Qi. Qi (pronounced as 'chi') is the life energy. This energy must flow freely around the body. If it gets blocked, there will be an imbalance in the body and that will be the cause of the different diseases and other health conditions.

According to the theory of Traditional Chinese Medical (TCM), the energies in the environment, those outside the body will affect everything that is inside the body.

This is a concept not new even to the modern western world. For instance, when it gets too cold and people do not protect themselves from the wind, there is a very huge possibility that one will suffer from cough and colds.

However, the western and eastern worlds approach to dealing with the problem is fairly different. For the latter, it is providing balance back to the body with the help of Shiatsu and other alternative modes of holistic treatment.

Like most Oriental form of healing, Shiatsu does not just adhere to the principle of Qi. It also believes that this life energy goes through certain channels in the body that correspond to the various organs or organ systems. These are the Meridians.

The Shiatsu Meridians

The more complex component of Shiatsu which must be learned is the various meridians. These are the channels in which the energy course through.

The Meridian theory is not just used in Shiatsu but also in other alternative forms of healing – especially if it originated in the East – such as Reflexology and Acupuncture.

Shizuto Masunaga, the developer of the Zen Shiatsu, has identified 12 meridians in the body. Most of these run from the head towards the lower back and / or the limbs (arms and legs). The others are situated in specific areas only.

These twelve meridians are not the actual organs. These only correspond to or symbolize certain organs or organ systems in the body. What Shiatsu does is to direct the energy towards those organs through these channels.

These meridians symbolize the following:
- Lung
- Large Intestine
- Stomach
- Spleen and Pancreas
- Heart
- Small Intestines
- Bladder
- Kidney
- Heart Governor
- Triple Heater
- Gall Bladder
- Liver

Some schools or styles of Shiatsu will have more meridians in their list. However, the twelve basic ones are included in the set all the time.

Acu-points in Shiatsu

The meridians are considered as the principal channels so, besides acting as the conduit of energy, the meridians have several dots or tsubos running through it. These individual dots are very similar to the acupressure and acupuncture points.

These tsubos are the parts of the meridians which may get blocked causing the disruption in the flow of energy and the imbalance or the health condition in the organ that it symbolizes.

With twelve various meridians (or more, for others), there are hundreds of these acu-points. Traditionally speaking, there are 364. Fifty of those are used frequently. Besides the tsubos, there are ashi points, the local areas where energy is actually blocked.

Besides being the points which are to be manipulated, the tsubos and ashis are used for diagnosis too. If these are swollen, painful or discolored, then there may be something wrong with the organ that the meridian or the actual point corresponds to.

Chapter IV - Styles of Shiatsu

Shiatsu was developed from different oriental healing methods from Japan and its neighboring countries. In the earlier part of the 20th century, when Tamai Tempaku came up with this form of massage therapy, he really had no idea that it would become so famous worldwide.

Today, Shiatsu comes in different forms and styles. The first two types which have been discussed earlier – the Zen Shiatsu and Namikoshi System – are the most popular of all. This is possibly because the two integrated science into it – something which has never been done before that.

This chapter will be about the different styles of Shiatsu, from the more traditional ones which are now recognized as modes of medical treatment in Japan and elsewhere in the world to those which have recently cropped up.

Namikoshi System

Tokujiro Namikoshi's Shiatsu journey started when he and his family moved to Hokkaido when he was seven years old and his mother started complaining of knee pain. Since there was no village doctor, he was the one who treated his mother by putting pressure on and rubbing the affected part.

After his success in making his mother feel well, he started learning Amma massage. Soon, he started integrating anatomy and physiology in what he has learned and made the Shiatsu massage more effective. Tokujiro Namikoshi is the one who founded the Japan Shiatsu Institute in the '40s.

Zen Shiatsu

This type of Shiatsu was developed by Shizuto Masunaga who is a psychologist. After his medical studies, he pursued Shiatsu under the tutelage of Namikoshi. He also adheres to Namikoshi's idea of incorporating age old Eastern healing methods (the Qi and the meridians in the body) with Anatomy, Physiology and Neurology.

Zen Shiatsu is very similar to Namikoshi's System except that it focuses more on psychological disorders. Shizuto Masunaga, its founder, is a psychologist. He integrated the ancient theories of pressure points and neurology in this form of Shiatsu.

Tsubo Therapy

Besides Masunaga and Namikoshi, Katsusuke Serizawa is another noteworthy individual when it comes to Shiatsu. He focused not just on the meridians but also on the tsubos, the individual points which run across the channels. Acupressure Shiatsu, a form of holistic therapy which combines Acupressure and Shiatsu, is actually derived from Serizawa's Tsubo Therapy.

Barefoot Shiatsu

Shizuko Yamamoto developed this and calls it as Macrobiotic Shiatsu as well. Although Yamamoto abides by the original principles set by his predecessors, he also believes that there is more to this if complete healing must be achieved.

For instance, Yamamoto supports a healthy and natural lifestyle which includes good diet, eating medicinal foods, enough rest and sleep and even the right breathing. Assessment is also very important for the diagnosis of the health condition of an individual. This should include visual, verbal and even touch.

Ohashiatsu

Developed by Wataru Ohashiatsu, this is a gentler, more nurturing type of Shiatsu. Besides the general principle, he put importance on the rapport between the giver of the massage and the receiver. He believes that the only way there will be healing is if there is good synergy between the two.

Tao Shiatsu

This is started by Ryokyu Endo. He believes that both the patient and the practitioner should reap the benefits of Shiatsu. Endo also did research on how Shiatsu should go with the rapid changes of the society and the environment so that it will continue to be an effective healing method.

Although he still stuck to the traditional spirit of Shiatsu but introduced various elements such as the 24 meridians instead of the original 12, the Super Vessel Specific Tsubos and improved Shiatsu diagnosis among others.

Watsu

This is also known as Water Shiatsu. Harold Dull, the man behind this style, mastered this in the '80s. He applied the general principles of Shiatsu on water and added stretches in the massage. Dull believes this to be more effective since, while the patient is floating, there is no stress on the vertebrae.

Quantum Shiatsu

Pauline Sasaki is the brainchild of this Shiatsu style. This focuses on the 'Energetic Body' which is more than just the physical form. From the term itself, this is influenced by Quantum Physics and how the theory of relativity can help with the process of healing. The biggest difference of Quantum Shiatsu from the rest is that it does not include Qi or the meridians anymore.

Jin Shin Do

Among all the Shiatsu styles, Ji Shin Do was developed by a non-Japanese - Iona Marsaa Teeguarden. Besides pressure on acu-points, this also incorporated body focusing techniques. This mind and body approach helps with both the physical and emotional state of an individual.

Chapter V - Reaping the Benefits of Shiatsu

Ever since Shiatsu was first introduced to the public in Japan, it has already garnered a lot of praise from the people who have tried and reaped its benefits. Even before the Japanese government credited this to be a legitimate medical treatment, some people in the western world, especially in the United States, have already tried this too.

All kinds of alternative medicine such as Acupuncture, Homeopathy, Reflexology, Iridology and even Shiatsu Massage practically share the same advantages.

100% Natural

Generally speaking, all alternative methods of treating diseases and other health conditions are natural. This, perhaps, is the reason why Shiatsu and these 'holistic' therapies are so popular today. After all, it's the time when the society has equated health with all-natural, 100% organic stuff.

Cheaper Now and in the Long Run

Squeezing out the juice of a lemon and adding a teaspoon of honey and drinking this for your cough would be less expensive than buying a bottle of cough syrup. This is one of the greatest benefits of going for alternative medication and therapies

If we are talking about going to the doctor to have your muscles and bones rehabilitated versus going for a deep tissue massage, maybe you would be spending less with the latter than the former.

Of course, one will hear the argument that Shiatsu, at $100 or so per hour's session, is just as expensive.

However, when one computes everything that may be spent on traditional medical treatment such as staying in a hospital overnight, medical testing and diagnostic fees, the remuneration of your doctor, the actual therapy, all the medication prescribed to you which must be bought and so many more, then it is possible that alternative modes of treatment is, indeed, less pricey.

No Adverse, Side Effects

Compared to taking in loads of pills, capsules, syrups or getting injected with really painful medications, choosing to get an hour's worth of massage is not just relaxing, you can be sure that you would not have to suffer through really irritating adverse and side effects.

Those are just the benefits of alternative medicines and therapies as a whole. If we are talking about Shiatsu, specifically, you will be amazed at the various advantages which one can enjoy.

Relaxation

The most obvious thing which Shiatsu really does is help one relax. Like most massage therapies, this is done in a warm, quiet, and soothing environment. This sort of ambience will definitely add so much to the actual pressing, rubbing and tapping on your tight and pained muscles.

Relief from Pain

Shiatsu, similar to most massage therapies, has been proven to alleviate the pain sensation. One of the explanations here is that massage tends to remove one's thoughts from pain probably because it provides such pleasure.

Besides that, Shiatsu relieves muscle tension which is one of the most probably causes of pain after injuries such as strains and sprains. Besides that, massage also improves circulation. Because of that, the overall movement of the various muscles will be made better as well.

Prevention of Diseases

Although some medical experts will dispute the concept of Shiatsu being a healing therapy by itself, massage can aid in preventing various diseases. Since manipulation of muscles all over the body will improve the circulation of blood, lymph and oxygen, the immune system will also be strengthened.

Chapter VI - How is Shiatsu Done?

Shiatsu, just like other massages, is a systematic process. However, it is quite similar to the medical methodologies. Apart from the usual things that are done by a masseuse in a regular massage for relaxation, it starts with a short interview followed by some sort of diagnostic examination before the actual treatment begins.

Interview and Diagnosis

At times, the person who needs a Shiatsu massage knows exactly what they want to achieve. There are other people who have no idea what is wrong with them – just that there is something wrong – and they want to try the massage.

Besides a short interview wherein the practitioner can build a good rapport with his or her patient, this is also the chance for the practitioner to have an idea regarding the health condition of the patient.

Examination of the different body parts will follow. The arms, legs, abdomen and back are usually checked for 'softness', 'hardness' and pain. Although the muscles of the whole body may still be manipulated, the problem area will be focused on for treatment.

Finding the Meridians

Since the principle of Shiatsu puts emphasis on the Qi and its flow through the channels, it would be the meridians that the practitioner would have to look for first.

The practitioner would usually run his fingers over the regions where the meridians supposedly are and feel for any irregularities like stiffness. Through various types of manipulation, the knots in that area will be loosened, allowing the energy to course through properly.

Rubbing, tapping and applying pressure on the area of the channel itself and /or the surrounding tissues are usually done for Shiatsu. The duration and the intensity may vary throughout the procedure.

Working on the Actual Massage

The position of the patient during Shiatsu may differ depending on what the patient really need. They could be asked to lie down on a soft but flat surface or sit down with a straight back on a chair.

Usually, the 'patient' is asked to lie on his stomach first. Using the palms and the base of the hand, knead the soles going up to the legs, buttocks, lower back and up to the shoulders.

After that, the thumbs will be used to knead the back of the head going back down the body in circular motions. Remember that more pressure must be placed on the 'tight' spots. If the knotted muscles feel too big or too tight, the area of the massage will be bigger as well. Usually, more time will be put on that region as well.

Allowing the 'patient' to rest after the whole massage is very important. The massage will last for an hour or so. Usually, the whole rubdown will last for forty-five minutes. The other 15 minutes will be for rest.

What Actually Happens Inside the Body During Shiatsu

After the massage has been completed and the energy is allowed to flow through the meridians once more, healing will commence.

The healing will be accompanied, almost immediately, by a great sense of wellbeing. This is because the pain sensation as well as feelings of stress will be obliterated.

The function of the lymph and circulatory system will also be improved. Because of this, the metabolites and other toxins stuck in the body will be excreted.

Another system which will improve in function would be the nervous and endocrine system. Because of the hormones which will be released, the 'patient' will feel happier, stronger and will have the ability to deal with the challenges in his or her life.

This is basically the essence of holistic therapy – treating the disease in the physical level and helping the individuals emotionally and psychologically as well.

What to Do Pre and Post Shiatsu

Both patients and practitioners must prepare for the procedure. This is very important so that the experience will be beneficial for both the giver and the receiver of Shiatsu massage.

Unlike other massages, essential oils aren't really needed for this. Although a private and peaceful environment is a must, incorporating music and 'oriental' décor is not really that important.

The masseuse should do some relaxation exercises so that he or she is at a certain level of tranquility as well. Since Shiatsu is all about Qi and its movement around the environment, it is very possible that the stress and negativity that the person is feeling may be transferred to the patient.

For people who will undergo the procedure, the preparation is not that complicated. As much as possible, the clothing to be worn should be soft and loose. Gym pants and t-shirts made of cotton would be perfect for this.

The patient should eat a good meal – but not a too heavy one. Drinking alcoholic beverages and eating fatty or salty foods are a huge no-no before and after Shiatsu.

Doing strenuous activities before and after the procedure is also not allowed. One will not be able to reap the total benefits if one is exhausted, after all.

There are other things which you may have to do before you do go through the process. Certain practitioners may have specific requirements from their patients. It would be best to ask them first so that you would not be surprised once you are there.

Chapter VII - The Side of Shiatsu Practitioners Don't Mention

Like most things, especially when it is our body and overall health that is on the line, it would be better to know both the pros and cons every single time. Shiatsu may very well be one of those miraculous healing methods when you hear a practitioner advertise it.

Obviously, they would not include the negative side of Shiatsu when they are trying to sell the service. But for your information and to help you with your decision making in whether to or not to undergo this procedure, here are some of the disadvantages, risks and contraindications of this massage therapy.

The Disadvantages of Shiatsu

One of the biggest problems that some people complain of regarding Shiatsu – especially the kind used as healing therapy – is that one session costs a lot. On an average, a session that lasts for an hour with a licensed practitioner may cost about $70.

Unfortunately, it will take more than one session to actually achieve wellness, if, as mentioned earlier, the goal is for treatment and not just for relaxation. Worse, not all health insurance policies cover this kind of therapy.

The other disadvantages of Shiatsu may not be too problematic for some. For instance, there are individuals who are not too comfortable getting almost naked or being touched by people they are not familiar with.

Another thing which some people do not really like about Shiatsu is that a session takes quite long. Compared to taking a pill for pain, which takes just about a second or so, Shiatsu massage for treatment will last for an hour to an hour and a half.

Shiatsu and the Possible Risks

Shiatsu massage also poses some risks for those who undergo it. Although these are not common and are carefully being prevented, cases of injuries after the massage have been reported.

Muscle soreness which may last for a few days and bruising are the major complaints of some people – especially if the masseuse pressed on the muscles too hard.

More often than not, these types of 'accidental' injuries are due to lack of practice in the part of the masseuse. It is very important, therefore, to choose someone who is not merely licensed but has been in the business for some time already.

Contraindications: Are You Even Allowed to Undergo Shiatsu?

Do take note that any kind of massage, including Shiatsu, has contraindications. This basically means that people who have certain diseases or are in some special health condition should not undergo Shiatsu.

Here is a list of the contraindications of Shiatsu massage:

- Fractures
  It would be best to wait until the fractures have healed completely.
- Open wounds and burns
- Rashes
  This may be due to allergic reactions. Psoriasis, although it is not a hypersensitivity reaction, is not allowed as well due to the breaks in the skin.
- Fungal infections
- Swelling on the skin
- Varicosities
- Hyperthermia or fever
- Viral or Microbial Infections
- Contagious skin diseases
  Besides the fact that the skin is broken and is not allowed, do not put the practitioner in danger. This includes chicken pox measles and shingles.

Fortunately, those who have the conditions listed above, all they really need to do is wait until the problem has cleared. There are some people who really should not undergo Shiatsu massage especially if they have the following medical conditions:

- Severe nerve damage
- Severe Osteoporosis

- ○ Cancer of the blood like Leukemia
- ○ Diabetes, especially uncontrolled types

Women with high risk pregnancies are also not allowed to undergo Shiatsu, or any massage for that matter. This may cause hemorrhaging and even miscarriage.

According to oncologists, it would be best if individuals with any type of cancer turn down Shiatsu massage. However, some massage practitioners and experts claim that it is alright as long as there manipulation is veered from the tumor.

In the case of Leukemia and other blood cancers, it is absolutely not allowed since the cancer cells will spread even faster around the body since the circulation will be improved by massage.

Chapter VIII - Shiatsu as an Adjutant Therapy

In Japan, Shiatsu massage is already a legitimate medical procedure since it was mandated by their government in the 60s.

One of the reasons why this became quite popular in the Western world is because of famous celebrities, rich socialites and politicians. Marilyn Monroe was the first one who tried the famous Namikoshi Shiatsu.

Today, there are so many medical practitioners who accept Shiatsu as an effective medium for relaxation and relief from certain symptoms, especially pain. However, there are still arguments whether this can be a stand-alone therapy to treat certain diseases or if traditional medical procedures and medications are still needed.

Proven Effects of Shiatsu

Although there are some experts who will adhere to the fact that Shiatsu is effective but only as an adjutant therapy to other modes of treatment, a lot of them agree that it can do so much in terms of relieving stress, improving one's sense of wellbeing and helping one to have a good night's sleep.

Research and Scientific Studies

Today, various hospitals, clinics and other medical facilities around the world are also quite interested with how Shiatsu works and its effects. Numerous researches and studies have been made to see if it will work, not just in the alleviation of symptoms, but also with diseases that do not have long-term and permanent treatment.

Here is a list of the different diseases which are currently being tested in relation to the effectiveness of Shiatsu as a mode of treatment, whether adjutant or stand-alone:

- AIDS and HIV
- Alzheimers
- Anxiety
- Arthritis and Other Joint Problems
- Asthma
- Autism
- Back Problems
- Cancer
- COPD
- Dementia
- Depression
- Diabetes
- Drug and Substance Abuse
- Fibromyalgia
- Migraines and Headaches
- Cardiac Problems
- Hysterectomy
- Irritable Bowel Syndrome
- Insomnia and other Sleep Problems
- Mental Illnesses
- Menstrual Problems
- Multiple Sclerosis
- Musculoskeletal Problems
- Panic Attacks
- Paralysis
- Parkinson's Disease
- Schizophrenia
- Sciatica
- Stroke

If you are suffering from any of those listed above and are thinking about giving Shiatsu a try, it would be best that you read as much about this. Numerous websites and Shiatsu societies on the internet may have information regarding this.

Besides doing your own research, it is essential that you consult with your doctor first. Working with your doctor is very important in this case, especially if there are no sufficient tests made.

Chapter IX - Shiatsu Massage Training

Working as a massage therapist specializing in Shiatsu is quite lucrative. As of the moment, one can earn as much as $200 for just an hour by performing this procedure. But of course, learning Shiatsu massage would be profitable. It is beneficial, not just for you, but for your family members and friends as well.

Naturally, one will have to undergo training and certification to be allowed to do Shiatsu massage.

Cost, Duration and Training Modules

If you do enroll in a Shiatsu institute, expect that you will study Anatomy and physiology, pathophysiology of diseases and the contraindications of those diseases.

Since this is Shiatsu, you will need to learn all about the Meridians and the specific tsubos or pressure points. In addition to that, you have to learn a bit about Chinese medicine and Shiatsu massage techniques specifically the Namikoshi System, Anma and Zen Shiatsu.

The duration of these programs will last from 300 hours to 700 hours, depending on what you really want to specialize.

For those who are serious about getting trained in Shiatsu and are thinking about working as a masseuse, one will have to spend as much as six to twelve thousand dollars for the whole course.

Schools for Shiatsu Training

In the mid-20th century, the Japan Shiatsu Institute was founded by Namikoshi, a forerunner in this Oriental alternative mode of healing. If you are quite serious about learning all about this and training to be a Shiatsu masseuse, then studying in that school would be advantageous for you.

Today, there are over dozens really good schools which you can enroll in. You do not have to go to Japan to be knowledgeable and skilled in Shiatsu. Since this is a very popular type of massage, every country in the world would surely have a training institute as well.

Going online would be one of the most certain ways to find a good school for Shiatsu learning and training.

www.ingramcontent.com/pod-product-compliance
Lightning Source LLC
Chambersburg PA
CBHW070245290526
45789CB00004B/1772